JUICING FOR COLD AND FLU

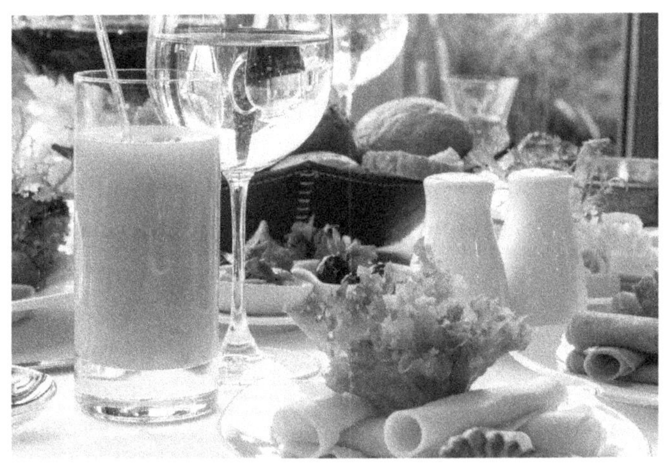

UNLOCK THE HEALING POWER OF JUICES TO COMBAT COLD AND FLU

CAMILA.C.HILL

TABLE OF CONTENT

1. Introduction

As someone who has experienced the misery of catching a cold or flu multiple times, I understand the frustration and discomfort that comes along with these illnesses. It wasn't until I discovered the power of juicing that I began to find true relief and prevention from these seasonal ailments.

Juicing for cold and flu has become my go-to strategy for boosting my immune system and accelerating my recovery. The beauty of juicing lies in its ability to deliver an abundance of nutrients directly to my body in a concentrated and easily digestible form. With just a simple glass of freshly extracted juice, I can provide my body with a plethora of vitamins, minerals, and antioxidants that work together to strengthen my immune system and combat pesky viruses.

One of the key elements in my cold and flu-fighting juices is the inclusion of vitamin C-rich ingredients. Citrus fruits like oranges and grapefruits, along with leafy greens like kale and spinach, have become staples in my recipes. These ingredients not only provide a generous dose of immune-boosting vitamin C but also offer other essential nutrients such as vitamin A and folate.

Additionally, I have discovered the incredible anti-inflammatory properties of ingredients like ginger and turmeric. These powerful roots have been used for centuries to alleviate symptoms associated with colds and flu. Incorporating them into my juices not only helps reduce inflammation but also provides natural pain relief and aids in soothing a sore throat.

Another remarkable benefit of juicing for cold and flu is the ability to target specific symptoms. For instance, when faced with nasal congestion, I turn to a blend of pineapple and eucalyptus, which helps clear my sinuses and relieve pressure. When coughing becomes my constant companion, a soothing blend of honey, lemon, and chamomile provides relief and comfort.

Juicing has not only become a tool for my recovery but also an essential part of my daily routine to prevent falling victim to these seasonal illnesses. I make sure to incorporate a variety of immune-boosting fruits, vegetables, and herbs into my daily juices to keep my body strong and resilient.

In conclusion, juicing for cold and flu has transformed my approach to these illnesses. It has become a powerful ally in my defense against viruses, providing me with the necessary nutrients to boost my immune system and alleviate symptoms.

From prevention to recovery, the natural goodness of freshly extracted juices has become my secret weapon in the battle against cold and flu.

a. The benefits of juicing for cold and flu relief

Juicing for cold and flu relief offers a multitude of benefits that can help alleviate symptoms and strengthen the immune system. Here are some key advantages:

1. Nutrient Powerhouse: Juicing allows you to consume a concentrated amount of essential nutrients in a highly bioavailable form. Fruits and vegetables are abundant in vitamins, minerals, and antioxidants that are crucial for supporting the immune system and fighting off viruses.

2. Immune System Boost: Certain ingredients, such as citrus fruits, berries,

and leafy greens, are known for their immune-boosting properties. Juicing allows you to easily incorporate these ingredients into your diet, providing your body with a robust defense against cold and flu viruses.

3. Quick Absorption: When you juice fruits and vegetables, you remove the fiber, making the nutrients more readily available to your body. This means that the vitamins and minerals are quickly absorbed into your bloodstream, providing immediate nourishment and support to your immune system.

4. Anti-Inflammatory Properties: Many fruits and vegetables used in juicing, such as ginger, turmeric, and leafy greens, possess excellent anti-inflammatory properties. Inflammation is a common symptom of colds and flu, and reducing it can help alleviate discomfort and promote healing.

5. Hydration: Staying hydrated is crucial for combating cold and flu symptoms.

Juicing offers a delicious and refreshing way to hydrate your body while also providing essential nutrients. Hydration helps to thin mucus, soothe sore throat, and maintain overall well-being.

6. Soothing Sore Throat: Juices made with ingredients like honey, lemon, and ginger have a soothing effect on a sore throat. These ingredients possess natural antibacterial properties and can help alleviate pain and discomfort while providing immune-boosting benefits.

7. Tailored Symptom Relief: With juicing, you can create specific recipes to address your individual symptoms. For example, adding ingredients like pineapple, eucalyptus, and mint can help clear nasal congestion, while a blend of honey, lemon, and herbs can provide relief from cough and chest discomfort.

8. Overall Well-being: Juicing is not only beneficial for cold and flu relief but also for promoting general wellness. Consuming a variety of fruits, vegetables, and herbs through juicing ensures that your body receives a wide range of nutrients, supporting overall health and vitality.

Incorporating juicing into your routine can provide relief from cold and flu symptoms, strengthen your immune system, and enhance your overall well-being. It is a natural and effective way to support your body's fight against these common illnesses.

b. Understanding the immune system and its importance

Understanding the immune system and its importance is crucial in recognizing how to support and optimize its function. Here's an overview:

The immune system is a sophisticated network of cells, tissues, and organs that collaborate to protect the body from detrimental pathogens, including bacteria, viruses, and fungi. Its main role is to identify and eliminate these invaders while maintaining a balance to prevent excessive reactions and damage to healthy cells.

The immune system consists of two main components: innate immunity and adaptive immunity. Innate immunity serves as the body's first line of defense and provides a general, non-specific response to pathogens. It includes physical barriers like the skin and mucous membranes, as well as immune cells like phagocytes, natural killer cells, and inflammation-inducing cytokines.

Adaptive immunity, on the other hand, is a specific and tailored response that develops over time. It involves specialized immune cells called T and B lymphocytes, which produce antibodies and memory cells. This component allows the immune system to remember and recognize specific pathogens it has encountered before, leading to a faster and more efficient response upon subsequent exposure.

The importance of the immune system goes beyond protecting us from common illnesses. It plays a vital role in preventing infections, maintaining overall health, and even defending against certain forms of cancer. A robust immune system is essential for optimal well-being at all stages of life.

However, various factors can negatively affect immune function, such as poor nutrition, chronic stress, lack of sleep, sedentary lifestyle, and exposure to environmental toxins. These factors can weaken the immune response and increase susceptibility to infectious diseases.

To support the immune system, adopting healthy lifestyle habits is crucial. This includes consuming a balanced and nutrient-rich diet, engaging in regular physical activity, managing stress levels, getting adequate sleep, maintaining proper hygiene practices, and avoiding harmful substances like tobacco and excessive alcohol consumption.

Additionally, certain nutrients, such as vitamins A, C, D, E, and minerals like zinc and selenium, play essential roles in immune function. Including a diverse range of fruits, vegetables, whole grains, lean proteins, and beneficial fats in your diet can help provide these immune-boosting nutrients.

Understanding the immune system's importance empowers individuals to take proactive steps in maintaining their health. By adopting a holistic approach that addresses lifestyle factors and includes immune-supporting practices, individuals can strengthen their immune system and enhance their body's ability to ward off infections and maintain optimal well-being.

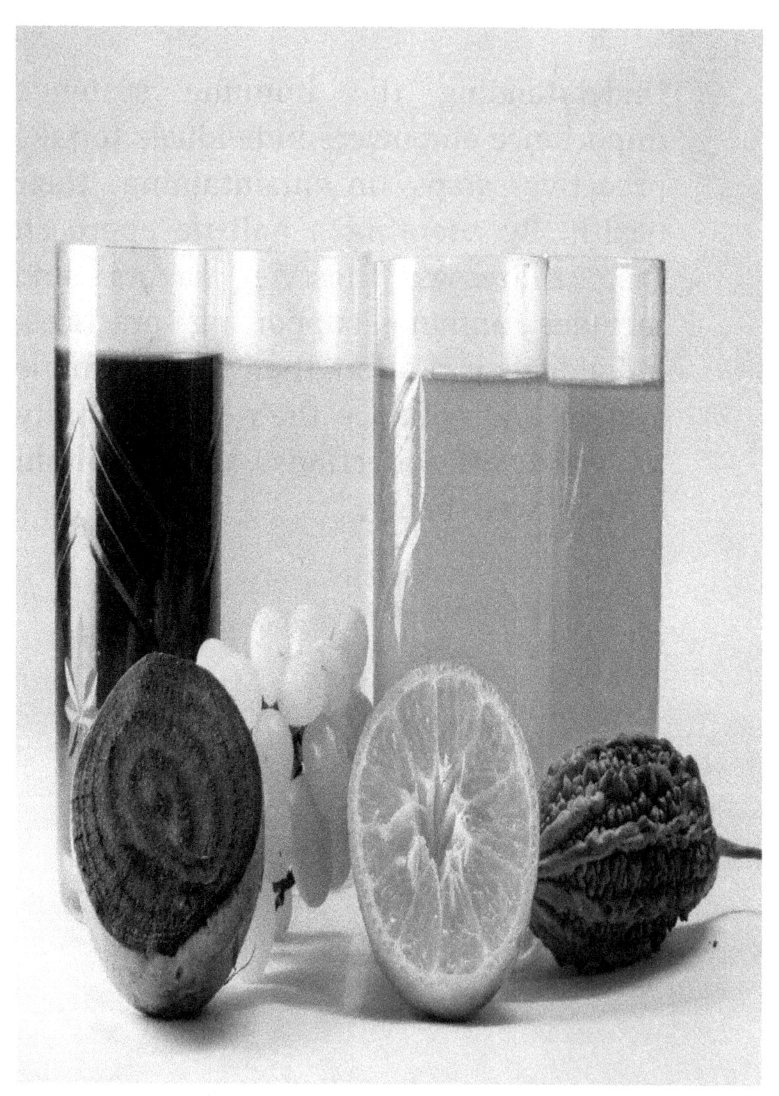

2. The Basics of Juicing

Juicing has gained significant popularity as a convenient and effective way to incorporate a wide range of fruits and vegetables into our diets. Here are the basics of juicing:

1. Equipment: To start juicing, you'll need a juicer or a high-powered blender. Juicers extract the juice from fruits and vegetables while leaving behind the fibrous pulp, while blenders blend the whole ingredients, including the fiber.

2. Ingredients: Choose a variety of fresh fruits, vegetables, herbs, and spices to create flavorful and nutrient-rich juices. Some popular options include leafy greens (spinach, kale, Swiss chard), citrus fruits (oranges, grapefruits, lemons), berries (blueberries, strawberries), root vegetables (carrots, beets), and herbs/spices (ginger, turmeric, mint).

3. Preparation: Wash all the ingredients thoroughly to remove any dirt or pesticides. Remove any peels, pits, or tough stems as needed. For juicers, cut the ingredients into smaller pieces that will fit into the juicer's feed chute. For blenders, you can leave the ingredients in larger chunks.

4. Juicing Process: For juicers, feed the prepared ingredients into the juicer, following its instructions. The juice will be collected in one container, while the pulp will be expelled into another. For blenders, add the ingredients along with some water or a liquid of your choice (e.g., coconut water, almond milk) and blend until smooth. You may need to strain the blended mixture through a nut milk bag or fine-mesh sieve to remove excess fiber.

5. Combining Flavors: Experiment with different flavor combinations to find the ones you enjoy. You can start with simple combinations like apple and spinach or be more adventurous with ingredients like beet, ginger, and orange. Remember that some ingredients may have stronger flavors, so adjust the amounts to your taste preferences.

6. Consumption: Freshly made juices are best consumed immediately to retain maximum nutritional value. However, if needed, refrigerate them in an airtight container for up to 24-48 hours. It's important to note that the vibrant colors of fruits and vegetables may oxidize over time, leading to a change in taste and nutrient content.

7. Cleanup: Pay attention to the cleaning process, as juicers and blenders can have several parts to disassemble and clean. Read the manufacturer's instructions for

proper cleaning and maintenance to ensure longevity and good performance of your equipment.

8. Variations: Aside from traditional juicing, you can also explore other options like smoothies (including the fiber) or using juiced ingredients in recipes for salads, soups, or even popsicles.

Remember that juicing should complement a well-rounded diet and not replace whole foods altogether. It can be an excellent way to boost your daily intake of fruits and vegetables, but it's essential to incorporate a variety of foods in their whole form as well.

By understanding the basics of juicing and getting creative with flavor combinations, you can enjoy the benefits of nutrient-rich juices and explore a world of delicious and healthy options.

a. Choosing the right juicer

Choosing the right juicer can make a significant difference in your juicing experience, efficiency, and the quality of the juice you produce. When choosing a juicer, there are several factors that should be taken into consideration.

1. Type of Juicer: There are several types of juicers available in the market. The main types are:

Centrifugal juicers are widely available and offer a cost-effective option for juicing. They work by grating the produce and extracting juice through centrifugal force. They are fast but may generate heat, which can slightly reduce the nutritional value of the juice.

b. **Masticating Juicers** (also known as Cold Press or Slow Juicers): These juicers use a slow grinding or chewing motion to extract juice. They are known for maintaining the highest nutritional value in the juice as they produce less heat and minimize oxidation. They are generally more expensive but yield higher quality juice with better juice extraction efficiency.

c. Citrus Juicers: These juicers are designed specifically for citrus fruits like oranges, grapefruits, and lemons. They are simple and affordable, ideal for those who primarily juice citrus fruits.

2. Speed and Efficiency: Consider how quickly you want to juice and the volume of juice you plan to make. Centrifugal juicers are generally faster, making them suitable for those with limited time. Masticating juicers are slower but offer better juice extraction efficiency, particularly with leafy greens or hard and fibrous vegetables.

3. Noise Level: Centrifugal juicers tend to be louder due to their high-speed spinning motion, while masticating juicers operate at a slower speed, producing less noise.

4. Cleaning and Maintenance: Some juicers have more parts and are more complex to clean, while others are easier to disassemble and clean. Consider your willingness and time commitment for cleaning when choosing a juicer.

5. Budget: Set a budget based on your needs and preferences. Juicers can range in price from affordable to high-end, depending on the type and brand.

6. Desired Juice Quality: If you prioritize maximum nutrient retention, a masticating juicer is generally recommended. If you primarily juice fruits and don't mind a slightly lower

nutrient content, a centrifugal juicer may be sufficient.

7. .Take into account the dimensions and storage needs of the juicer in relation to the available space.Some juicers are compact and easily fit on countertops, while others may require more space.

8. Reviews and Reputation: Read reviews and consider the reputation of the juicer brand to ensure reliability, durability, customer service, and customer satisfaction.

Ultimately, the right juicer will depend on your personal preferences, budget, and juicing goals. Consider these factors to choose a juicer that fits your specific needs and enhances your juicing experience.

b. Selecting the best produce for cold and flu prevention

Selecting the right product can play a crucial role in boosting your immune system and potentially preventing colds and flu. Here are some fruits and vegetables known for their immune-boosting properties:

1. Citrus Fruits: Oranges, lemons, grapefruits, and limes are rich in vitamin C, which is known to enhance immune function and help fight off infections.

2. Berries: Blueberries, strawberries, raspberries, and blackberries are packed with antioxidants and vitamin C, which can support immune function.

3. Leafy Greens: Spinach, kale, Swiss chard, and other leafy greens are

excellent sources of vitamins A, C, and E, as well as various antioxidants. Consuming freshly squeezed juices can aid in boosting your immune system.

4. Garlic: Garlic has antimicrobial and immune-enhancing properties. It contains compounds like allicin that can help fight infections and support immune health.

5. Ginger: Ginger has anti-inflammatory and antioxidant properties and may help boost the immune system. It can be added to teas, juices, and various dishes.

6. Bell Peppers: Bell peppers, especially red bell peppers, are rich in vitamin C, which can support immune function.

7. Turmeric: Turmeric contains curcumin, a compound with anti-inflammatory and antioxidant properties

that may enhance immune response and reduce the risk of infections.

8. Cruciferous Vegetables: Broccoli, cauliflower, Brussels sprouts, and cabbage are all members of the cruciferous family and are packed with vitamins, minerals, and antioxidants that can support overall health and immune function.

9. Kiwi: Kiwis are a good source of vitamin C, vitamin E, and other essential nutrients that can support the immune system.

10. Papaya: Papaya is rich in vitamin C, as well as a digestive enzyme called papain, which has anti-inflammatory and immune-supporting properties.

It's important to note that consuming a variety of fruits and vegetables is key to getting a wide range of nutrients that support immune health. Furthermore, while these foods can contribute to a healthy immune system, they cannot solely prevent colds or the flu. Good hygiene practices, adequate sleep, stress management, regular physical activity, and a well-balanced diet overall are important in maintaining a strong immune system.

Always consult with a healthcare professional for personalized advice and if you have specific dietary considerations or health conditions.

c. Tips for juicing at home

Juicing at home can be a great way to incorporate more fruits and vegetables into your diet and enjoy the benefits of fresh and nutritious juice. Consider these helpful tips to assist you in getting started:

1. Choose fresh and high-quality produce: Select fresh, ripe, and organic fruits and vegetables whenever possible. This ensures that you get the best flavor and nutritional value in your juice.

2. Wash your produce: Thoroughly wash all your fruits and vegetables before juicing to remove any dirt, pesticides, or bacteria. Use a produce wash or a mixture of water and vinegar for optimal cleanliness.

3. Balance your ingredients: Create a well-rounded juice by combining different types of produce. Mix leafy greens with fruits, add some herbs or spices for flavor, and consider including a variety of colors to get a wider range of nutrients.

4. Start with smaller quantities: If you're new to juicing, start with smaller quantities of ingredients until you get

accustomed to the flavors. You can gradually increase the amount as you experiment and find combinations that you enjoy.

5. Experiment with flavors: Don't be afraid to be adventurous and experiment with different flavor combinations. Add a piece of ginger for a zing, some lemon for freshness, or a handful of mint for a burst of flavor. Be creative and find what suits your taste buds.

6. Drink your juice immediately: Freshly made juice is best consumed immediately to retain the maximum nutritional value and freshness. However, if you need to store it for a short period, do so in an airtight container in the refrigerator. Keep in mind that the juice might lose some nutrients and freshness over time.

7. Use a variety of fruits and vegetables: To get a wide spectrum of nutrients, vary

the types of fruits and vegetables you juice. This ensures that you get a mix of vitamins, minerals, antioxidants, and phytonutrients from different sources.

8. Clean your juicer thoroughly: After each use, disassemble your juicer and clean all the parts properly. This prevents build-up of residue, maintains performance, and ensures the longevity of your juicer.

9. Incorporate the pulp: Instead of discarding the pulp, consider using it in other recipes. You can add it to baked goods, soups, smoothies, or even use it as compost for your garden.

10. Listen to your body: Pay attention to how your body responds to different ingredients. Some people may have sensitivities or allergies to certain fruits or vegetables. In case you encounter any

negative reactions, it is advisable to seek advice from a healthcare professional.

Remember, juicing should complement a well-balanced diet and not replace whole foods. It's important to consume a variety of fruits, vegetables, whole grains, lean proteins, and healthy fats to ensure you get all the essential nutrients your body needs.

Juicing can be a fun and creative way to enhance your nutritional intake and enjoy a wide range of flavors. Experiment, have fun, and tailor your juices to your own preferences and wellness goals.

3. Essential Nutrients for Cold and Flu Prevention

When it comes to cold and flu prevention, it's important to ensure that you're getting a balance of essential nutrients that support a healthy immune system. Give priority to these essential nutrients:

1.Renowned for its immune-boosting properties, Vitamin C is an essential nutrient to prioritize. It helps stimulate the production of white blood cells, which are essential in fighting off infections. Excellent sources of vitamin C include citrus fruits, strawberries, kiwi, bell peppers, and leafy greens.

2. Vitamin D: Vitamin D plays a crucial role in immune function. It is often obtained through sunlight exposure, but it can also be found in fatty fish (salmon,

mackerel), fortified dairy products, egg yolks, and mushrooms.

3. Zinc: Zinc has antiviral properties and supports immune cell function. Incorporate zinc-rich foods like oysters, beef, poultry, legumes, nuts, and seeds into your diet.

4. Omega-3 Fatty Acids: Omega-3 fatty acids help reduce inflammation and support immune function. Good sources include fatty fish (salmon, sardines, mackerel), walnuts, flaxseeds, and chia seeds.

5. Probiotics: Probiotics promote a healthy gut microbiome, which plays a role in immune response. Yogurt, kefir, sauerkraut, and other fermented foods are great sources of probiotics.

6. Antioxidants: Antioxidants help protect cells from damage caused by free

radicals and support immune function. Colorful fruits and vegetables like berries, leafy greens, tomatoes, and carrots are rich in antioxidants.

7. Garlic: Garlic has immune-boosting properties and contains compounds that have antiviral and antimicrobial effects.

8. Ginger: Ginger has anti-inflammatory and antioxidant properties that can support immune health. It can be consumed through teas, juices, or added to various dishes.

9. Turmeric: Curcumin, the active compound in turmeric, has anti-inflammatory and antioxidant properties. It has been found to enhance immune response and reduce the risk of infections.

10. Water: Staying hydrated is essential for overall wellness and immune

function. Water helps flush toxins out of the body and supports the proper functioning of all its systems.

Remember that a well-rounded diet, regular exercise, adequate sleep, stress management, and good hygiene practices are also vital in maintaining a strong immune system and preventing colds and flu. If you have specific dietary considerations or health conditions, it's best to consult with a healthcare professional or registered dietitian for personalized advice.

a. Vitamin C-rich juices for boosting immunity

Below are some delicious and vitamin C-rich juice combinations to help boost immunity:

1. Citrus Blast:
   - 2 oranges

- 1 grapefruit
- 1 lemon

2. Green Sunshine:
   - 2 oranges
   - 1 cup spinach
   - 1 kiwi
   - ½ cucumber

3. Berry Boost:
   - 1 cup strawberries
   - 1 cup raspberries
   - 1 orange
   - ½ lemon

4. Tropical Immunity:
   - 1 mango
   - 1 cup pineapple
   - 1 orange
   - ½ lime

5. Citrus Carrot Delight:
   - 2 oranges
   - 2 carrots

- ½ lemon
- 1 inch ginger root

6. Pomegranate Power:
   - 1 cup pomegranate seeds
   - 1 orange
   - 1 apple
   - ½ lemon

7. Citrus Ginger Zing:
   - 2 oranges
   - 1 grapefruit
   - 1 inch ginger root

8. Kiwi Lime Refresher:
   - 4 kiwis
   - ½ lime
   - Handful of mint leaves

9. Pineapple Citrus Splash:
   - 2 cups fresh pineapple
   - 1 orange
   - 1 lemon
   - ¼ cup fresh mint leaves

10. Watermelon Citrus Cooler:
   - 2 cups watermelon
   - 1 orange
   - ½ lime
   - Handful of fresh basil leaves

Feel free to adjust the quantities of ingredients based on your taste preferences and the juicing capacity of your equipment. Remember to wash all fruits and vegetables thoroughly before juicing and enjoy these vitamin C-rich juices as part of a balanced diet.

b. Antioxidant-packed juices for fighting off infections

Here are some antioxidant-packed juice combinations to help fight off infections:

1. Berry Blast:

- 1 cup blueberries
- 1 cup strawberries
- ½ cup raspberries
- ½ cup blackberries

2. Beet Cleanser:
- 1 beetroot
- 2 carrots
- 1 apple
- ½ lemon
- 1-inch ginger root

3. Green Antioxidant Kick:
- 2 cups spinach
- ½ cucumber
- 2 celery stalks
- Handful of parsley
- ¼ pineapple

4. Citrus Turmeric Elixir:
- 2 oranges
- 1 grapefruit
- ½ lemon
- 1-inch turmeric root

-Include a pinch of black pepper to improve the absorption of turmeric.

5. Mango Carrot Immunity Booster:
    - 1 mango
    - 2 carrots
    - ½ orange
    - ½ lime
    - 1 tablespoon chia seeds (rich in antioxidants)

6. Green Apple Detox:
    - 2 green apples
    - 1 cucumber
    - 1 cup kale or spinach
    - ½ lemon
    - Small handful of mint leaves

7. Pineapple Ginger Spice:
    - 2 cups fresh pineapple
    - 1 apple
    - 1-inch ginger root

8. Cabbage Calm:

- ½ small green cabbage
- 2 carrots
- 1 orange
- ½ lemon
- Handful of fresh basil leaves

9. Purple Power:
   - 1 cup purple grapes
   - 1 cup blueberries
   - ½ cup raspberries
   - ½ cup pomegranate seeds

10. Tomato Antioxidant Mix:
   - 2 ripe tomatoes
   - 1 red bell pepper
   - 1 carrot
   - ¼ small red onion
   - Handful of fresh basil leaves

Remember to adjust the quantities based on your preferences and equipment capacity. These antioxidant-packed juices can be a great addition to your diet to support your immune system and help fight off infections.

c. Immune-boosting herbs and supplements to add to your juices

Adding immune-boosting herbs and supplements to your juices can provide an extra nutritional punch. Here are some options to consider:

1.Renowned for its immune-boosting properties, Echinacea is a widely recognized herb. It can help activate and enhance the function of immune cells. Look for echinacea extract or tincture and follow the recommended dosage instructions.

2. Astragalus: Astragalus is an herb widely used in traditional Chinese medicine known for its immune-

enhancing effects. It can help support immune system function and reduce the risk of infections. Look for astragalus extract or tincture and follow the recommended dosage instructions.

3. Elderberry: Elderberry has been used for centuries to support the immune system. It contains antioxidants and compounds that can help shorten the duration of cold and flu symptoms. Look for elderberry syrup or extract and follow the recommended dosage instructions.

4. Ginseng: Ginseng is an adaptogenic herb that can help enhance the immune system. It has been shown to have immunomodulatory effects and may improve the body's defense against infections. Look for ginseng extract or tincture and follow the recommended dosage instructions.

5. Containing curcumin, turmeric possesses antioxidant and anti-inflammatory properties that aid in maintaining a healthy immune response.. Add a teaspoon of turmeric powder or a slice of fresh turmeric root to your juices.

6. Ginger: Ginger has anti-inflammatory and antioxidant properties that can support immune health. It also has antimicrobial properties that can help fight off infection. Add a thumb-sized piece of fresh ginger root to your juices.

7. Probiotics: Probiotics can help support a healthy gut microbiome, which in turn supports immune function. Consider adding a high-quality probiotic supplement or a spoonful of probiotic powder to your juices.

Remember to consult with a healthcare professional or herbalist before adding any herbs or supplements to your routine, especially if you have any underlying health conditions or are taking medications. They can provide personalized advice and dosage recommendations based on your specific needs.

4. Recipes for Cold Relief

Here are some soothing and comforting juice recipes that can provide relief during a cold:

1. Citrus Soother:
    - 2 oranges
    - 1 lemon
    - 1-inch ginger root
    - 1 tablespoon honey (optional)

2. Ginger Turmeric Tonic:
    - 1-inch ginger root
    - 1-inch turmeric root (or 1 teaspoon turmeric powder)

- 2 carrots
- 1 orange
- ½ lemon

3. Immune-Boosting Trio:
    - 1 apple
    - 2 cups spinach
    - 1 cup pineapple
    - ½ lemon

4. Pineapple Mint Elixir:
    - 2 cups fresh pineapple
    - Handful of mint leaves
    - 1 tablespoon honey (optional)

5. Carrot-Orange Glow:
    - 2 oranges
    - 3 carrots
    - ½ lemon
    - 1-inch ginger root

6. Green Cold Fighter:
    - 2 cups spinach
    - 1 cucumber

- 2 celery stalks
- ½ cup parsley
- 1 green apple

7. Berry Soothing Blend:
    - 1 cup strawberries
    - 1 cup blueberries
    - ½ cup raspberries
    - ½ cup blackberries
    - 1 orange

8. Pineapple-Ginger Fizz:
    - 2 cups fresh pineapple
    - 1-inch ginger root
    - ½ lime
    - Sparkling water (to taste)

9. Turmeric-Carrot Comfort:
    - 2 carrots
    - 1 orange
    - 1-inch turmeric root (or 1 teaspoon turmeric powder)
    - ½ lemon
    - 1 tablespoon honey (optional)

10. Cooling Herbal Blend:
   - 1 cucumber
   - Handful of fresh mint leaves
   - Handful of fresh basil leaves
   - 1 cup coconut water

Remember to adjust the quantities based on your preferences and juicing capacity. These recipes can provide soothing relief during a cold, thanks to their nutrient content and potential anti-inflammatory properties. Additionally, staying hydrated and consuming warm soups and herbal teas can also contribute to your comfort and recovery.

a. Ginger and Turmeric Wellness Shot

Certainly! Here's a recipe for a Ginger and Turmeric Wellness Shot:

Ingredients:
- 1-inch ginger root
- 1-inch turmeric root (or 1 teaspoon turmeric powder)
- Juice of 1 lemon
- Add a dash of black pepper to optimize the absorption of turmeric.
- For added sweetness, you may include a teaspoon of honey or maple syrup, if desired.

Instructions:
1. Peel the ginger root and turmeric root (if using fresh roots).
2. Juice the ginger and turmeric root using a juicer or grate them finely and squeeze out the juice using a cheesecloth or strainer.
3. In a small bowl, combine the ginger and turmeric juice with the lemon juice. If using turmeric powder, add it to the mixture instead.

4. Add a dash of black pepper to the mixture. The presence of black pepper can boost the absorption of curcumin, the active component found in turmeric.

5. For some sweetness, you can add honey or maple syrup and stir until well combined.

6. Pour the mixture into a shot glass or small glass.

7. Take the shot in one go, or sip on it slowly if you prefer.

Note: Ginger and turmeric have a strong and spicy taste, so adjust the ingredients based on your preference. You can also dilute the shot with some water or mix it into your favorite juice for a milder flavor.

Ginger and turmeric are both known for their anti-inflammatory and immune-boosting properties, making this shot a great way to support your overall wellness. Enjoy!

b. Citrus Blast Juice for Vitamin C Boost

Absolutely! Here's a recipe for a Citrus Blast Juice that will give you a vitamin C boost:

Ingredients:
- 2 oranges
- 1 grapefruit
- 1 lemon
- 1 lime
- Optional: 1-inch ginger root (for added flavor and immune support)

Instructions:
1. Peel the oranges, grapefruit, lemon, and lime, removing the outer rinds but leaving as much of the white pith as possible since it contains beneficial nutrients.

2. Cut the fruits into pieces that can fit into your juicer.

3. If you're using ginger, peel and slice the ginger root.

4. Juice the oranges, grapefruit, lemon, lime, and ginger root (if using), one at a time, in your juicer.

5. Once all the fruits have been juiced, give the juice a good stir to combine the flavors.

6. Pour the juice into a glass and enjoy it immediately to retain maximum freshness and nutritional value.

This Citrus Blast Juice is packed with vitamin C, a powerful antioxidant that supports immune health and aids in collagen production. The combination of oranges, grapefruit, lemon, and lime provides a refreshing and tangy flavor profile. The ginger root can add a hint of spiciness and provide additional immune-boosting benefits.

Feel free to adjust the ingredients to your taste preferences and add ice cubes if you prefer a chilled juice. It's a great way to start your day or boost your immune system whenever you need an extra dose of vitamin C!

c. Immune-Boosting Green Juice

Certainly! Here's a recipe for an immune-boosting green juice:

Ingredients:
- 2 cups spinach
- 1 cucumber
- 2 celery stalks
- ½ cup parsley
- 1 green apple
- Juice of ½ lemon
- Optional: 1-inch ginger root (for added flavor and immune support)

Instructions:

1. Wash all the ingredients thoroughly.

2. Cut the cucumber and celery into smaller pieces that can fit into your juicer.

3. Core the green apple and cut it into quarters.

4. If using ginger, peel and slice the ginger root.

5. Juice the spinach, cucumber, celery, parsley, green apple, lemon juice, and ginger (if using), in your juicer one at a time.

6. Once all the ingredients have been juiced, give the juice a good stir to combine the flavors.

7. Pour the juice into a glass and enjoy it immediately for maximum freshness and nutritional value.

This immune-boosting green juice is packed with nutrients and antioxidants to support your immune system. Spinach, cucumber, celery, parsley, and green apple provide a wealth of vitamins, minerals, and phytonutrients. The addition of lemon juice adds a refreshing tang, while ginger offers a hint of spiciness and additional immune-boosting benefits.

Please feel free to modify the ingredients and their quantities according to your personal taste preferences. You may also want to add ice cubes if you prefer a chilled juice. Enjoy this flavorful and nourishing green juice as part of your healthy routine to give your immune system a boost!

5. Recipes for Flu Recovery

a. Anti-inflammatory Beet and Berry Blend

Certainly! Here's a recipe for an anti-inflammatory Beet and Berry Blend:

Ingredients:
- 1 small beetroot, peeled and diced
- 1 cup of assorted berries, such as blueberries, strawberries, and raspberries.
- 1 cup of almond milk or any plant-based milk of your choosing.
- 1 tablespoon chia seeds
- 1 tablespoon of honey or maple syrup (if desired, for added sweetness).

Instructions:
1. Add the diced beetroot, mixed berries, almond milk, chia seeds, and optional sweetener (if desired) to a blender.
2Blend on a high speed until the mixture is smooth and fully combined. . If the

consistency is too thick, you can add more almond milk to reach your desired consistency.

3. Taste the mixture and adjust the sweetness by adding more honey or maple syrup if needed.

4. Pour the blend into a glass or jar.

5. Optionally, you can let the mixture sit in the refrigerator for a few minutes to allow the flavors to meld and the chia seeds to thicken the mixture.

6. Serve and enjoy your nutritious and anti-inflammatory Beet and Berry Blend!

Beets are known for their anti-inflammatory properties, as they contain antioxidants such as betalains that can help reduce inflammation in the body. Mixed berries are also rich in antioxidants, providing additional anti-inflammatory benefits. Chia seeds are a great source of omega-3 fatty acids, fiber, and antioxidants, which can further support inflammation reduction.

This blend is not only delicious but also packed with beneficial nutrients. Enjoy it as a refreshing and nutritious snack or as a part of your daily routine to support your overall well-being.

b. Flu-Fighting Pineapple and Kale Juice

Certainly! Here's a recipe for a flu-fighting Pineapple and Kale Juice:

Ingredients:
- 2 cups kale
- 1 cup fresh pineapple chunks
- 1 cucumber
- 1 green apple
- 1-inch piece of ginger
- Juice of 1 lemon

Instructions:
1. Wash all the ingredients thoroughly.

2. Tear the kale leaves into smaller pieces.

3. Cut the cucumber and green apple into smaller chunks.

4. Peel and slice the ginger into smaller pieces.

5. Juice the kale, pineapple chunks, cucumber, green apple, ginger, and lemon juice in your juicer, one at a time.

6. Once all the ingredients have been juiced, give the juice a good stir to combine the flavors.

7. Pour the juice into a glass and enjoy it immediately for maximum freshness and nutritional value.

This flu-fighting juice contains ingredients that provide immune-boosting properties. Kale is packed with vitamins A and C, which help support a healthy immune system. Pineapple is a rich source of bromelain, an enzyme known for its anti-inflammatory properties. Cucumber adds hydration and helps to balance the flavors, while green apple adds sweetness. The addition of ginger provides a spicy kick and additional immune-boosting benefits.

You are welcome to make adjustments to the ingredients and amounts to suit your personal taste preferences.. You can also add ice cubes to make it a chilled juice. Enjoy this flavorful and nutritious Pineapple and Kale Juice to support your immune system during flu season!

c. Healing Herbal Infusions for a Speedy Recovery

1. Ginger and Lemon Infusion:
- Ingredients: 1-inch piece of fresh ginger, sliced; Juice of 1 lemon; Honey (optional)
- Instructions: Boil a cup of water and add the sliced ginger. Let it steep for

about 5 minutes. Strain the ginger and add the lemon juice. Optionally, sweeten with honey. Sip on this soothing infusion to help relieve congestion, boost digestion, and provide a dose of vitamin C.

2. Chamomile and Peppermint Infusion:
- Required Ingredients: 1 tablespoon of dried chamomile flowers; 1 tablespoon of dried peppermint leaves; Optional: Honey for sweetening.
- Instructions: Boil a cup of water and add the dried chamomile flowers and peppermint leaves. Let it steep for about 10 minutes. Strain the herbs and add honey if desired. Chamomile helps calm and relax the body, while peppermint can help soothe an upset stomach and improve digestion. This infusion is perfect for promoting relaxation and aiding in recovery.

3. Echinacea and Elderberry Infusion:

- Ingredients: 1 tablespoon dried echinacea root or leaves; 1 tablespoon dried elderberries; Honey (optional)
- Instructions: Boil a cup of water and add the dried echinacea root or leaves and elderberries. Let it simmer for about 15 minutes. Strain the herbs and add honey to taste. .Echinacea and elderberry are renowned for their ability to strengthen the immune system.This infusion can help support the immune system and speed up recovery from illness.

4. Turmeric and Cinnamon Infusion:
- Ingredients: 1 teaspoon ground turmeric; 1 teaspoon ground cinnamon; 1 tablespoon honey; 1 cup plant-based milk (such as almond milk)
- Instructions: In a small saucepan, heat the plant-based milk over medium heat. Add the turmeric and cinnamon. Stir well to combine and let it simmer for a few minutes. .Take the mixture off the heat

and incorporate honey to add sweetness.Turmeric and cinnamon both have anti-inflammatory properties that can support the body's healing process.

Choose the herbal infusion that aligns with your specific needs and preferences. .It is important to seek guidance from a healthcare professional if you have any pre-existing medical conditions or are currently taking medications.Enjoy these healing herbal infusions as part of your recovery regimen for a speedy and healthy recovery!

6. Incorporating Cold-Fighting Superfoods

a. Adding garlic, ginger, and turmeric to your juices

can provide numerous health benefits. These three ingredients are renowned for their potent anti-inflammatory and antioxidant properties, as well as their immune-boosting and digestion-enhancing effects. Here are some benefits of including garlic, ginger, and turmeric in your juices:

1. Anti-inflammatory properties: All three ingredients have powerful anti-inflammatory properties that can help reduce inflammation in the body. Chronic inflammation has been linked to several health conditions, including heart disease, diabetes, and certain types of cancer. Including garlic, ginger, and

turmeric in your juices can help combat inflammation and promote overall health.

2. Immune-boosting effects: Garlic, ginger, and turmeric are known for their immune-boosting abilities. They contain compounds that can enhance the function of immune cells, helping to strengthen your immune system and protect against infections and diseases.

3. Digestive health: Ginger and turmeric are beneficial for digestion. Ginger can help relieve nausea, bloating, and indigestion, while turmeric can support a healthy gut by reducing inflammation and promoting the growth of beneficial gut bacteria. Adding these ingredients to your juices can aid in digestion and improve overall gut health.

4. Antioxidant properties: Garlic, ginger, and turmeric are rich in antioxidants,

which help protect your cells from damage caused by harmful free radicals. Antioxidants can help reduce the risk of chronic diseases, slow down the aging process, and support overall well-being.

5. Flavor and aroma: Along with their health benefits, garlic, ginger, and turmeric can add a delicious flavor and aroma to your juices. They can create a zesty and unique taste that enhances the enjoyment of your juice.

When incorporating these ingredients into your juices, it's important to note that they have strong flavors that might not be everyone's preference. Start by using small amounts and gradually increase the quantity to suit your taste. Additionally, if you have any specific health concerns or are taking medications, it's advisable to consult with a healthcare professional before making significant changes to your diet.

b. Exploring the benefits of elderberry and echinacea

Elderberry and echinacea are two plant-based ingredients that have gained popularity for their potential health benefits. These two ingredients have several associated benefits:

Elderberry:
1. Immune support: Elderberry is well-known for its immune-boosting properties. It contains antioxidants that help strengthen the immune system and support its function, potentially reducing the severity and duration of colds and flu.
2. Cold and flu relief: Elderberry has been traditionally used to alleviate symptoms of the common cold and flu, such as cough, congestion, and sore throat.
3. Antioxidant activity: Elderberry is rich in antioxidants, specifically

anthocyanins, which protect cells from oxidative stress and damage caused by free radicals. Antioxidants have been associated with various health benefits, including reducing inflammation and promoting overall well-being.

4. Heart health: Some research suggests that elderberries may have positive effects on heart health. It may help lower cholesterol levels and support healthy blood pressure, reducing the risk of cardiovascular diseases.

Echinacea:

1. Immune support: Echinacea is widely used as a natural remedy for boosting the immune system. It stimulates the production and activity of immune cells, helping the body defend against infections such as the common cold, respiratory tract infections, and even urinary tract infections.

2. Anti-inflammatory properties: Echinacea contains compounds with

anti-inflammatory effects that can help reduce inflammation in the body. Inflammation is associated with many chronic conditions, and by reducing it, echinacea may provide additional health benefits.

3. Energy and vitality: Some studies suggest that echinacea may improve energy levels and promote overall vitality. It is believed that its immune-boosting effects contribute to enhanced overall well-being and energy levels.

Both elderberry and echinacea can be consumed in various forms, such as capsules, syrups, teas, and even incorporated into juices and smoothies. However, it's important to note that while these ingredients have been traditionally used and have shown promising results in some studies, more research is needed to fully understand their benefits and any potential interactions or side effects. As always, it's recommended to consult with a healthcare professional before adding any new supplements or ingredients to your routine, especially if you have any specific health conditions or are taking medications.

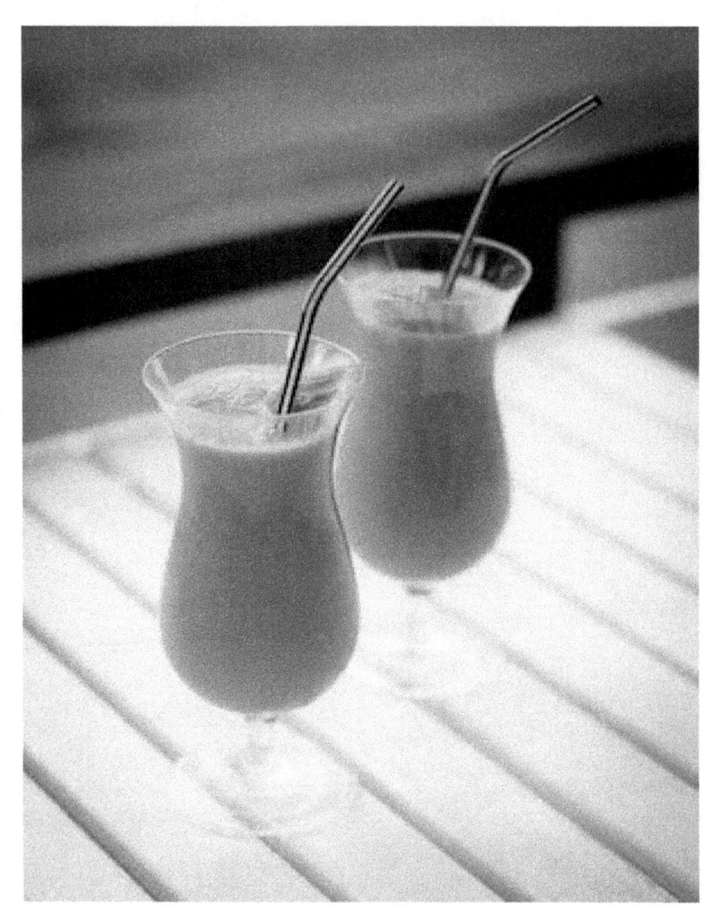

7. Juicing for Symptom Relief

a. Soothing sore throat with specific juice blends

When it comes to soothing a sore throat, certain juice blends can be helpful in providing relief and supporting the healing process. Here are a few juice combinations that you can try:

1. Lemon, ginger, and honey: Lemon is rich in vitamin C and has antimicrobial properties that can help ease the discomfort of a sore throat. Ginger has anti-inflammatory properties that can help reduce swelling and pain. Honey has soothing effects and can also help ease a sore throat. Combine the juice of half a lemon, a teaspoon of grated ginger, and a tablespoon of honey with warm water for a soothing drink.

2. Pineapple, cucumber, and mint: Pineapple contains bromelain, an enzyme that has anti-inflammatory properties

and may help reduce swelling and pain in the throat. Cucumber is hydrating and may provide relief. Mint can have a soothing effect on the throat. Juice some pineapple chunks, cucumber slices, and a few sprigs of fresh mint for a refreshing and throat-soothing blend.

3. Apple, pear, and chamomile: Apples and pears are gentle on the throat and can help provide hydration. Chamomile tea is known for its soothing properties and can help alleviate throat inflammation. Juice some apples and pears, and mix the juice with a cup of cooled chamomile tea for a soothing and comforting drink.

4. Carrot, orange, and turmeric: Carrots and oranges are high in vitamin C, which can support the immune system and promote healing. Turmeric has anti-inflammatory and antioxidant properties that may help reduce throat discomfort.

Juice a couple of carrots, an orange, and a teaspoon of turmeric for a nourishing juice blend.

Remember to drink these juices at room temperature or slightly warmed to avoid irritating the throat further. Additionally, it's important to note that these juice blends can provide relief but may not cure the underlying cause of a sore throat. If your symptoms persist or worsen, it's best to consult a healthcare professional for proper diagnosis and treatment.

b. Clearing nasal congestion with decongestant juices

When dealing with nasal congestion, decongestant juices can offer relief by providing hydration, vitamins, and compounds that can help alleviate the congestion. Here are a few juice combinations that may help clear nasal congestion:

1. Orange, lemon, and ginger: Oranges are rich in vitamin C, which can support the immune system and reduce inflammation. Lemons also contain vitamin C and have antimicrobial properties. Ginger has anti-inflammatory effects and may help relieve congestion. Juice some oranges, squeeze in the juice of half a lemon, and grate a teaspoon of ginger for a refreshing and decongestant blend.

2. Pineapple, cucumber, and mint: Pineapple contains an enzyme called bromelain that can help reduce swelling and congestion in the sinuses. Cucumber is hydrating and can help soothe the nasal passages. Mint has a cooling effect and may provide relief. Juice some pineapple chunks, cucumber slices, and a

few sprigs of fresh mint for a refreshing and decongestant drink.

3. Carrot, beetroot, and turmeric: Carrots are high in vitamin A, which can support the immune system, while beetroot is packed with antioxidants that can help reduce inflammation. Turmeric has anti-inflammatory and antimicrobial properties that may help relieve congestion. Juice some carrots, a small beetroot, and a teaspoon of turmeric for a nutrient-rich decongestant blend.

4. Tomato, celery, and garlic: Tomatoes contain antioxidants and vitamin C, which can help reduce inflammation. Celery has a high water content and can help keep the nasal passages hydrated. Garlic has antimicrobial properties that may assist in relieving congestion. Juice a few tomatoes, a couple of celery stalks, and a clove of garlic for a decongestant juice blend.

It's essential to drink plenty of fluids when dealing with nasal congestion, as hydration can help thin mucus and ease congestion. Additionally, steam inhalation, saline nasal rinses, and over-the-counter nasal decongestants or saline sprays can also be helpful adjuncts in relieving nasal congestion. If your symptoms persist or worsen, it's advisable to consult a healthcare professional for further evaluation and guidance.

c. Easing cough and chest discomfort with targeted recipes

When it comes to easing a cough and chest discomfort, certain recipes can be beneficial in providing relief and soothing the respiratory system. Here are a few targeted recipes that you can try:

1. Honey and herbal tea: Honey has soothing properties that can help alleviate cough symptoms, especially when combined with herbal teas known for their respiratory benefits. You can brew a cup of herbal tea, such as chamomile, peppermint, or ginger tea, and add a tablespoon of honey to it. Sip on this warm concoction to soothe your throat and relieve cough.

2. Turmeric milk: Turmeric contains curcumin, a compound with anti-inflammatory and antioxidant properties that may help ease chest discomfort and cough. Warm up a cup of milk (dairy or plant-based), add a teaspoon of turmeric powder, and optionally, a pinch of black pepper for better absorption of curcumin. Mix well and enjoy this comforting drink before bed.

3. Ginger and pear smoothie: Ginger has anti-inflammatory properties and may

help alleviate chest discomfort. Pears are rich in vitamins and antioxidants that can boost the immune system. Blend a ripe pear with a teaspoon of grated ginger, a squeeze of lemon juice, and a cup of water or almond milk. You can also add a tablespoon of honey or a dash of cinnamon for added flavor.

4. Homemade cough syrup: Create a homemade cough syrup by mixing together equal parts of honey, lemon juice, and coconut oil. Optionally, you can add a pinch of cayenne pepper for extra relief. Take a teaspoon of this syrup as needed to soothe your cough and reduce chest discomfort.

Remember, these recipes are intended to provide temporary relief and should not replace medical advice. If your cough persists or worsens, or if you have any underlying health conditions, it is recommended to consult a healthcare professional for proper diagnosis and treatment.

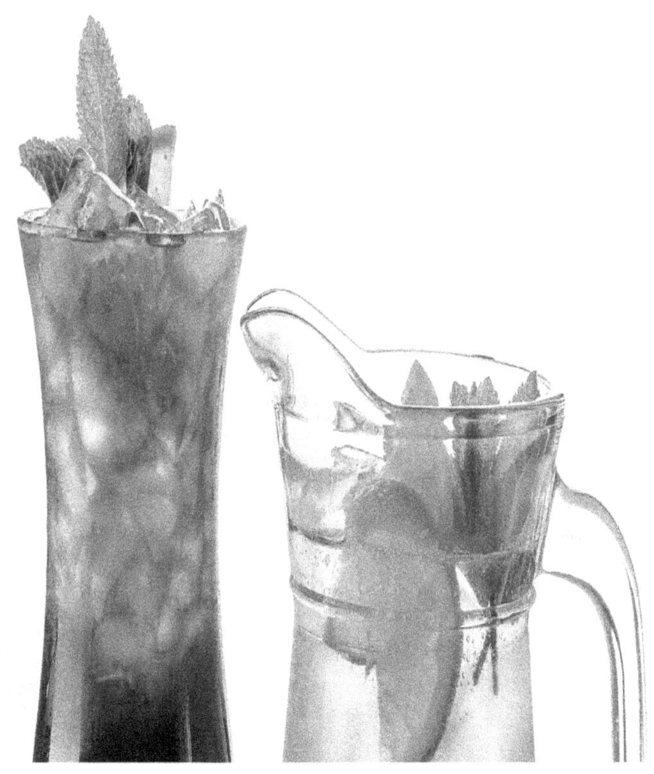

8. Lifestyle Tips for Cold and Flu Prevention

a. Building a strong immune system through proper nutrition and sleep

Building a strong immune system is crucial for overall health and prevention of illnesses. Proper nutrition and sufficient sleep play significant roles in supporting and boosting the immune system. Here are a few suggestions to enhance both:

1. Maintain a well-rounded diet by incorporating a multitude of fruits, vegetables, whole grains, lean proteins, and healthy fats into your meals. These foods offer crucial nutrients, vitamins, and minerals that help strengthen the immune system. Strive for a diverse array of colorful fruits and vegetables to maximize your intake of essential nutrients.

2. Increase intake of immune-boosting foods: Certain foods have immune-boosting properties, such as citrus fruits (rich in vitamin C), berries (abundant in antioxidants), garlic (anti-inflammatory and antimicrobial), ginger (anti-inflammatory), and yogurt (probiotics). Make it a habit to include these foods in your regular diet.

3. Stay hydrated: Drinking enough water helps flush out toxins and supports immune function. Aim for at least 8 glasses of water per day, or more if you are physically active or in a warm climate.

4. Prioritize sleep: Quality sleep is vital for immune health. .Strive to achieve a sufficient and uninterrupted sleep of 7-9 hours each night.Establish a regular sleep schedule and create a sleep-friendly

environment by keeping the room dark, quiet, and at a comfortable temperature.

5. Manage stress: Long-term stress has the potential to compromise the immune system's functionality. Practice stress management techniques like exercise, meditation, deep breathing, or engaging in hobbies you enjoy. Prioritize self-care activities to promote relaxation and reduce stress levels.

6. Limit processed foods and added sugars: Highly processed foods and excessive added sugars can contribute to inflammation and weaken immune function. Choose whole, unprocessed foods as your priority and reduce the consumption of sugary beverages, snacks, and desserts.

7. Maintain a healthy weight: Obesity can impair immune function. Sustain a healthy weight by incorporating a well-

balanced diet, engaging in regular physical activity, and practicing portion control.

8. Practice good hygiene: Wash your hands regularly, especially before eating or touching your face, to avoid the spread of germs. Proper hygiene helps prevent illnesses and supports a healthy immune system.

Remember that a healthy immune system is not solely dependent on nutrition and sleep. Regular exercise, avoiding smoking and excessive alcohol consumption, and getting recommended vaccinations are also important factors in maintaining a strong immune system. If you have specific health concerns, it is always best to consult a healthcare professional for personalized advice.

b. Hygiene practices to minimize exposure to cold and flu viruses

To minimize exposure to cold and flu viruses, practicing good hygiene is crucial. Outlined below are crucial hygiene practices to adhere to:

1Practice frequent handwashing: Ensure to wash your hands thoroughly with soap and water for a minimum of 20 seconds, particularly prior to meals, after using the restroom, and following exposure to public environments. . If soap and water are unavailable, use hand sanitizer with at least 60% alcohol.

2. Avoid touching your face: Viruses can enter your body through your eyes, nose, and mouth. Refrain from touching your

face, particularly with unwashed hands, to reduce the risk of transmission.

3. Cover your mouth and nose: Use a tissue or your elbow to cover your mouth and nose when coughing or sneezing. By promptly disposing of used tissues and subsequently washing your hands, you can effectively mitigate the transmission of respiratory droplets that may harbor viruses.

4. Use disposable items when sick: If you are ill with a cold or flu, use disposable tissues, napkins, or paper towels instead of reusable handkerchiefs. This prevents the buildup and transfer of viruses.

5. Clean and disinfect frequently-touched objects and surfaces: Regularly clean and disinfect surfaces such as doorknobs, light switches, countertops, and electronic devices. Use household

disinfectants or diluted bleach solution for effective disinfection.

6. Stay away from sick individuals: If possible, avoid close contact with individuals who are visibly sick with cold or flu symptoms. By implementing these measures, you can minimize the chances of coming into contact with the virus and reduce your risk of exposure.
7. Practice respiratory etiquette: If you have symptoms of a cold or flu, stay home from work or school to prevent the spread of the virus to others. Follow the guidelines and recommendations of your healthcare provider or local health authorities.

8. Maintain a healthy lifestyle: A healthy lifestyle supports a strong immune system.To maintain good overall health and bolster your immune system, it is important to consume a well-balanced diet, engage in regular physical activity,

ensure an adequate amount of sleep, and effectively manage stress levels.. A robust immune system can better defend against viruses.

Remember, while these hygiene practices can reduce the risk of exposure to cold and flu viruses, they are not foolproof. It is essential to stay informed about current guidelines from health authorities and follow any specific recommendations provided by healthcare professionals.

c. Exercises and stress reduction techniques for strengthening overall health

Exercises and stress reduction techniques are key components of maintaining overall health and well-being. Here are some examples:

1. Cardiovascular exercises: Engaging in aerobic exercises, such as brisk walking, jogging, swimming, or cycling, can improve cardiovascular health, strengthen the heart, and increase overall endurance. Aim for at least 150 minutes of moderate-intensity aerobic activity per week.

2. Strength training: Incorporating strength training exercises, like weightlifting or bodyweight exercises, helps build muscle strength, increases bone density, and improves overall physical function. Aim for two or more days a week of strength training targeting major muscle groups.

3. Yoga: Yoga combines physical poses, breathing techniques, and meditation to promote flexibility, balance, strength, and stress reduction. Regular practice of yoga enhances both physical and mental

well-being. Consider joining a yoga class or following online tutorials.

4. Pilates: Pilates focuses on core strength, flexibility, and body awareness. It involves controlled movements that target specific muscle groups. Pilates can improve posture, stability, and overall body strength. Join a Pilates class or try at-home workouts.

5. Mindfulness meditation: Mindfulness meditation involves focusing your attention on the present moment, accepting it without judgment. Regular practice can reduce stress, improve focus, and promote emotional stability. Begin with shorter sessions and gradually extend the duration over a period of time.

6. Deep breathing exercises: Deep breathing techniques, such as diaphragmatic breathing, can help reduce stress, lower blood pressure, and promote relaxation. Find a quiet space,

sit comfortably, and focus on slow, deep breaths, inhaling through your nose and exhaling through your mouth.

7. Tai Chi: Tai Chi is a low-impact exercise that combines gentle movements and deep breathing. This ancient Chinese practice improves balance, flexibility, and overall body coordination. You can consider joining a Tai Chi class or following instructional videos to learn and practice Tai Chi.

8. Outdoor activities: Spending time in nature, whether it's walking in a park, hiking, or gardening, can reduce stress levels, enhance mood, and improve overall well-being. Even a short time outdoors can have significant benefits.

It is crucial to seek advice from a healthcare professional before embarking on any new exercise routine, particularly if you have any pre-existing health conditions or concerns. Additionally, finding activities that you enjoy and incorporating them into your daily routine can help create a sustainable and enjoyable approach to improving overall health.

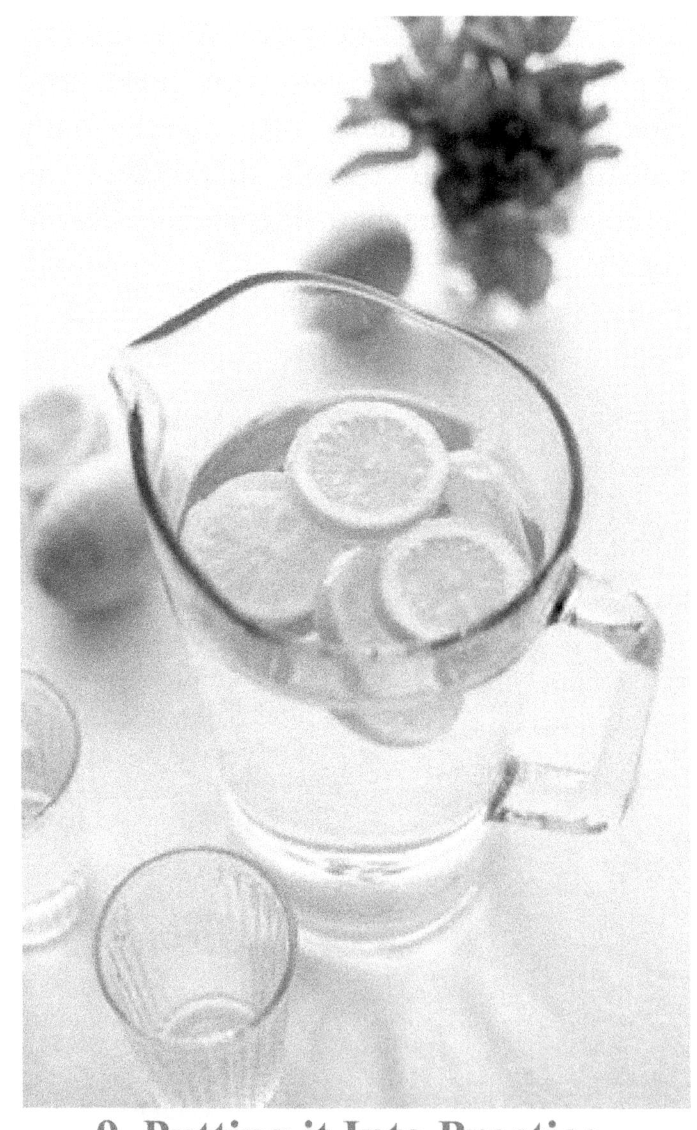

9. Putting it Into Practice

a. Creating a juicing routine for prevention and recovery

Creating a juicing routine can be a great way to incorporate nutrient-rich fruits and vegetables into your diet for prevention and recovery. Here are some tips for creating a juicing routine:

1. Choose a variety of fruits and vegetables: Opt for a diverse range of fruits and vegetables to maximize the nutrient content of your juices. Include leafy greens like spinach or kale, along with fruits like apples, oranges, berries, and carrots. Mix and match different ingredients based on your taste preferences.

2. Focus on immune-boosting ingredients: Include fruits and vegetables known for their immune-boosting properties. Citrus fruits like oranges and lemons are rich in vitamin C, which supports immune function. Ginger and

turmeric have anti-inflammatory properties, and leafy greens such as spinach and kale are packed with vitamins and minerals.

3. Incorporate hydration boosters: Add hydrating ingredients like cucumber or watermelon into your juices to ensure you stay well-hydrated. These ingredients also provide additional vitamins and minerals.

4. Experiment with superfoods: Consider adding superfoods like chia seeds, flaxseed, spirulina, or wheatgrass to your juices. These ingredients provide extra antioxidants, omega-3 fatty acids, or other health benefits. Start with small amounts and gradually increase as you find what works for you.

5. Maintain a balanced approach: While juicing can be beneficial, it's important to remember that whole fruits and

vegetables are also essential for the fiber they provide. Aim to consume whole fruits and vegetables alongside your juices to ensure you get the full range of nutrients and fiber that aid digestion and overall health.

6. Be mindful of portion sizes: Juicing can concentrate the natural sugars present in fruits, so be mindful of portion sizes to avoid excessive sugar intake. Aim for a balanced blend of fruits and vegetables to keep the sugar content in check.

7. Make it a regular habit: Incorporate juicing into your routine by setting aside specific times each day or week for preparation. It could be in the morning as a refreshing start to your day or as a mid-afternoon pick-me-up.To fully maximize the benefits of juicing, maintaining a consistent routine is essential.

8. Stay mindful of your individual needs: Everyone's nutritional needs may differ based on age, health conditions, and personal preferences. Consider consulting a healthcare professional or registered dietitian to tailor a juicing routine that suits your specific needs and goals.

Remember, while juicing can be a valuable addition to a healthy lifestyle, it should not replace balanced meals or be relied upon as the sole source of nutrition. It is important to maintain a varied and nutritious diet that includes a mix of whole foods alongside your juicing routine.

b. Incorporating juicing into your daily diet

Incorporating juicing into your daily diet can be a great way to boost your intake of fruits and vegetables and enhance your overall nutrition. Here are a few suggestions to assist you in integrating juicing into your daily schedule:

1. Start by investing in a good quality juicer: Choose a juicer that suits your needs and budget. There are various types available, including centrifugal juicers (fast and efficient), masticating juicers (slow and efficient), and citrus juicers (specifically for citrus fruits). Select one that aligns with your preferences and requirements.

2. Plan your juice recipes: Take some time to plan your juice recipes in advance. This will help you ensure that you have all the necessary ingredients on hand and can save you time in the morning. Explore different combinations of fruits, vegetables, and additional add-ins for variety and nutritional benefits.

3. Include a mix of fruits and vegetables: Aim for a balanced combination of fruits and vegetables in your juices. Vegetables like spinach, kale, cucumber, celery, and carrots are packed with essential nutrients, while fruits like apples, oranges, berries, and pineapples can add natural sweetness and flavor to your juices.

4. Experiment with flavors: Don't be afraid to get creative and experiment with different flavor combinations. You can add herbs like mint or basil, spices like ginger or turmeric, or even a splash of citrus juice to enhance the taste of your juices.

5. Consider timing: Choose the timing of your juices carefully. Drinking them in the morning can provide a fresh start to your day and can be a good replacement for processed breakfast options. However, you can also enjoy juices as a

mid-morning or afternoon snack, or even with meals.

6. Be mindful of portion sizes: While juices can be nutritious, it's important to be mindful of portion sizes, especially if you're watching your sugar intake. Stick to a reasonable serving size, usually around 8-12 ounces, and avoid consuming excessive amounts of juice in one sitting.

7. Don't forget the fiber: While juicing removes the fiber content from fruits and vegetables, it's important to ensure that you're still consuming fiber through other meals and snacks. Consider incorporating whole fruits, vegetables, and whole grains in your diet to maintain a balanced fiber intake.

8. Clean your juicer thoroughly: After each use, clean your juicer thoroughly to prevent the buildup of bacteria. Follow

the manufacturer's instructions for cleaning and make sure to disassemble all the parts and wash them with warm, soapy water.

Remember, juicing is a supplement to a healthy diet and should not replace whole foods. Aim to incorporate a variety of fruits, vegetables, whole grains, lean proteins, and healthy fats into your overall daily diet for optimal nutrition and well-being.

c. Tips for juicing on-the-go

Juicing on-the-go can be a convenient way to maintain a healthy diet, even when you have a busy schedule. Here are some tips to help you juice while you're on the move:

1. Pre-prepare ingredients: Preparing your fruits and vegetables in advance can save you time and make juicing on-the-

go easier. Wash, peel (if necessary), and chop your produce ahead of time. Portion them into individual servings and store them in airtight containers or reusable bags in the refrigerator.

2. Use a travel-friendly juicer: Invest in a portable juicer or blender that is designed for travel. Look for a compact and lightweight option that will be easy to carry around. You can find small, personal blenders or juicers that can be used with portable cups or bottles.

3. Pack your ingredients: If pre-cutting your produce isn't feasible, pack your fruits and vegetables along with a small cutting board and knife in a travel-friendly bag. Make sure to keep the perishable items cool with an ice pack or insulated bag.

4. Opt for single-serve containers: Use single-serve containers, such as mason

jars or reusable bottles, to store your juices. These containers are convenient to carry, and you can enjoy your juice directly from them. Ensure that the containers are leak-proof and seal tightly to avoid spills.

5. Juice in advance: If you have access to a juicer at home, consider juicing in bulk and storing the prepared juice in sealed containers in the refrigerator. This way, you can grab a bottle of juice when you're on-the-go and enjoy it whenever you need a quick nutrient boost.

6. Seek juice bars or cafes: When you're out and about, look for juice bars or cafes that offer freshly made juices. This can be a hassle-free way to get your juice fix without having to prep or carry your own equipment.

7. Choose travel-friendly ingredients: Select produce that can withstand being

stored for longer periods without spoiling. Apples, carrots, celery, citrus fruits, and firm vegetables like beets or cucumbers tend to travel well and stay fresh.

8. Stay hydrated: In addition to juicing, ensure you stay hydrated throughout the day by carrying a refillable water bottle. Hydration is essential for overall health, and water can complement your juicing routine by keeping you refreshed.

Remember to be mindful of food safety practices when juicing on-the-go. Keep your prepared juices refrigerated or in a cooler with ice packs if you're not consuming them immediately. Dispose of any leftover juices if they've been left unrefrigerated for an extended period or if you suspect any spoilage.

By planning ahead and making smart choices, you can enjoy the benefits of juicing even when you're away from home.

10. Conclusion

In conclusion, incorporating juicing into your routine can be a valuable tool for prevention and recovery from cold and flu symptoms. By selecting nutrient-dense fruits and vegetables, immune-boosting ingredients, and hydration enhancers, you can create powerful juices to support your immune system and overall health. Remember to maintain a balanced approach, consult with professionals if needed, and incorporate whole foods alongside your juicing routine. With mindful planning and a commitment to consistency, juicing can play a significant role in supporting your body's natural defenses against cold and flu viruses. Cheers to juicing for cold and flu prevention and recovery!